The Pocket Guide to Mouth and Dental Hygiene in Dementia Care

THE POCKET GUIDE to MOUTH and DENTAL HYGIENE in DEMENTIA CARE

Guidance for Maintaining Good Oral Health

DR DANIEL J. NIGHTINGALE

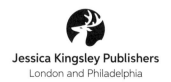

Jessica Kingsley Publishers
London and Philadelphia

First published in 2020
by Jessica Kingsley Publishers
73 Collier Street
London N1 9BE, UK
and
400 Market Street, Suite 400
Philadelphia, PA 19106, USA

www.jkp.com

Library of Congress Cataloging in Publication Data
A CIP catalog record for this book is available from the Library of Congress

British Library Cataloguing in Publication Data
A CIP catalogue record for this book is available from the British Library

ISBN 978 1 78775 130 9
eISBN 978 1 78775 131 6

Printed and bound in Great Britain

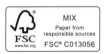

Contents

Introduction

Oral care in the senior population is no less important than in other age groups. For example, current statistics show that one in ten older adults die from aspiration pneumonia. This makes it the leading cause of death among this population. A contributing factor to aspiration pneumonia is poor oral hygiene and dental neglect (Manabe *et al.* 2015).

Many older people, those living with dementia and those experiencing mental health challenges face major issues with this area of self-care. There are many reasons for this, and they are addressed in the chapters that follow.

I have been a clinical dementia specialist since 2002 and a clinical hypno-psychotherapist working in the field of mental health since 2007. Working across both the UK and US, I am greatly concerned about the malignant impact that dental neglect has on both psychological and physical health. Unfortunately, in the UK, it isn't always easy finding and registering with an NHS dentist, and paying privately can be expensive. For example, a private dental exam costs £42, a full set of dentures around £554, a first initial consultation £53 and £60 for a cleaning. In the US, if you don't have dental insurance, treatment costs can be extensive, therefore many people may make dental care the least of their priorities. For example, a basic cleaning in Arizona, which should be done every six months (this may be every three if one experiences tooth or gum disease), costs approximately $100. In a state where benefits are not overly common or easily accessible, the reader can see how this would be a financial burden on someone living with dementia or mental illness.

Vulnerable people, whether children or adults, require as much support as possible with this area of self-care; this guide will assist in achieving that goal. It can be very challenging brushing an individual's teeth, especially if that person does not comprehend what is being done to them (a poignant reminder here that we should be supporting and doing *with* people and not *to* them). Visiting a dentist's office can increase the fear and anxiety levels of those living with dementia, severe clinical depression, schizoaffective disorder or other mental illness, and those with Down's syndrome and Alzheimer's disease. There are many other developmental disorders such as autism, and mental illnesses such as schizophrenia where meeting oral hygiene and dental care needs may require innovative approaches and interventions. The key to a successful outcome is to step outside our reality and into that of the person we are supporting.

In this guide, I will cover how poor dental and oral care impacts negatively on the individual; tips and tricks for optimal oral care; proactive oral and dental care; prioritizing oral care needs; how to spot oral disease; oral care and mental illness, and the positive dental experience. At the end of the book there are interactive case studies that involve the reader, and five common questions that are asked by those supporting the person through their particular journey.

The overall aim is to ensure that the reader is equipped with additional knowledge and skills to improve oral care and hygiene as well as dental treatment. Ultimately this will lead to enhanced quality of life through good physical and psychological health.

Dr Daniel J. Nightingale, PhD; RN;
ADHP (NC); ECCH; CHt, clinical dementia specialist
and clinical hypnopsychotherapist

CHAPTER 1

The Impact of Neglected Oral Hygiene

Although this chapter discusses the physical implications of poor dental and oral care, it is important first to consider the psychological issues that are likely to compound the existing journey of dementia, and the day-to-day effects of living with mental health challenges.

The three areas of concern here relate to body image, confidence and self-esteem. To demonstrate the malignant impact on these three areas of an individual living with dementia, I would like to introduce you to Anne (name changed to protect anonymity and adhere to doctor/patient confidentiality). Figure 1.1 illustrates how these three states of emotional being converged to add further challenges to an already vulnerable individual.

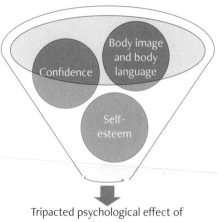

Tripacted psychological effect of
neglected oral hygiene

Figure 1.1: The tripacted model[1]

Anne was an 83-year-old lady living independently in the home she had shared with her husband for over 50 years. Sadly, he passed away approximately 12 months prior to Anne slipping on the ice and breaking one of her upper front teeth to such an extent that only a small piece of it remained intact. Though Anne was living with Alzheimer's disease, she continued to be a very proud lady, taking great pride in her appearance. She was sociable and very popular within the community, attending many functions throughout the week. After her fall, other members of the community noticed that she was beginning to go out less and less. Her son, who had recently become her power of attorney, had suggested this may be due to her dementia getting worse. However, her friends believed it was more to do with the damage to her

---

1   The tripacted model relates to the three major components (tri) that impact on a given issue (in this case, confidence, body image and body language, and self-esteem).

tooth, though Anne had not spoken with her son about it. His belief was that at her age nobody cared how she looked. However, he had not asked her about this.

I was asked to see her because the GP thought she may have clinical depression or that her reluctance to go out was due to progression of the Alzheimer's disease. From my initial interview, it was apparent that Anne was experiencing negative emotion, leading to malignant social psychology, within the three emotional states. Let's address each one as they affected her.

Body image is defined in psychology as a person's emotional attitudes, beliefs and perceptions of their own body. It has been defined as the multifaceted psychological experience of embodiment. As you can see by viewing the tripacted model in Figure 1.1, this was affecting not only Anne's body image, but her body language too. She didn't want to smile because of how it looked, therefore, her body language expressed an air of seriousness along with a closed personality. As we know, this was not Anne's true character. People's perception of her, based on this initial body language, was incorrect. She felt embarrassed to smile, which in turn meant she felt ugly, and as she put it, 'It makes me feel weird.'

Confidence is defined by the English Oxford Living Dictionary as a feeling of self-assurance arising from an appreciation of one's own abilities or qualities. In this situation, the change in Anne's body image and expression of body language was suppressing her confidence. During our consultation and spotlighting exercise, I discovered that her lowered confidence was the main reason she had not spoken to her son about how she was feeling. Her self-confidence was sinking fast.

Self-esteem relates to how one feels about oneself. In psychology, the term self-esteem is used to describe a person's overall sense of self-worth or personal value – in other words, how much you appreciate and like yourself. Anne had always felt good about herself. She was brought up to take pride in both her appearance and the way she looked. Now her self-esteem was at an all-time low, and she had even stopped looking in the mirror when getting ready for the day ahead. Therefore, her hair was not brushed properly, she had stopped applying make-up and had begun to look very unkempt.

Malignant social psychology is a term that was coined by the late Professor Tom Kitwood when he was referring to the overall impact of certain behaviours in care delivery that lead to a reduction in the individual's personhood. We can easily see from the above that Anne's personhood was beginning to disintegrate at a rapid rate.

Solution

First, I facilitated a discussion between Anne and her son. She was anxious about sharing her feelings with him as she didn't want to upset him, put him out or cause him any problems. I coached her through this challenge by utilizing a technique called 'empty chair therapy'. I encouraged Anne to imagine her son was sitting in a chair and she was able to express her feelings, needs and wishes in a structured, unthreatening manner. After doing this a few times, she felt ready to speak with her son Alan. I facilitated the meeting and, as she explained how she was feeling and the reasons for her withdrawal, Alan reached over and gave her a big hug! The following day, she was at the dentist's office beginning the process of having her broken tooth replaced. Over the weeks that followed, we all witnessed a return of the Anne everyone had grown to know and love.

When supporting people through their journey – whatever that journey may be – it is imperative that carers are familiar with the individual's personality, character and life story. We all have a responsibility to help maintain a person's identity, dignity and self-worth. Failure to do so results in diminished personhood and we, as caregivers, provide the nutrition that fuels disintegration of a fellow human being.

Neglected dental treatment and oral hygiene is never acceptable, and we will now see the physical impact of such neglect.

There is a well-known adage that says, 'Ignore your teeth and they'll go away.' That's exactly what happens when good oral hygiene practices are neglected. For patients living with dementia or other mental health challenges, maintaining good or even minimal levels of acceptable oral hygiene becomes an increasingly challenging task, yet a very important one.

The most significant dental health problems for dementia patients are caused by a deterioration in their ability to perform self-care oral health practices. This progressive neglect of good oral hygiene practices, like brushing teeth and gums, flossing, rinsing with recommended mouthwashes and cleaning dentures is due in part to a loss of the manual dexterity required for these tasks. Those living with dementia reach a point where they forget the need (or even how) to brush their teeth, gums or dentures. This neglect of oral hygiene unfortunately increases as the severity of dementia progresses.

These challenges put added demands on caregivers to assume the responsibility of maintaining good oral health in the people they are supporting. Caregivers need to assist and eventually completely take over good oral health practices.

The oral health complications of poor oral health are significant. They include:

- Loss of teeth

- Inflammation of the gums

- Halitosis

- Tooth ache

- Loose teeth

- Tooth or gum abscess

- Loss of ability to adequately chew food

- Difficulty swallowing.

When you have a healthy mouth, you can speak, smile, eat and drink. An unhealthy mouth means discomfort, severe pain and disease.

Good general health is about so much more than a nice smile and healthy teeth and gums, since the mouth is a primary entry point into the body. Poor oral health can have negative consequences throughout the entire body. Teeth that ache, gums that bleed and breath that smells are all indicators of poor oral health. Bacteria from the mouth can easily get into the bloodstream or lungs and spread infection and inflammation throughout the body.

Here are some common, yet serious, general health problems linked to poor oral health:

- Increased risk for heart disease. This means a greater chance of having a heart attack, stroke, hypertension or endocarditis (an infection of the heart's inner lining, usually involving the heart valves).

- Infected gums may release substances that kill brain cells. This can lead to memory loss and enhance dementia symptoms.

- Respiratory infections are caused when bacteria in the mouth are breathed into the lungs or travel through the bloodstream. This causes pneumonia, acute bronchitis or even chronic obstructive pulmonary disease. As mentioned in the Introduction, aspiration pneumonia, a leading cause of death among seniors, is exacerbated by poor oral hygiene.

- Gum disease can lead to high blood sugar levels, increasing the risk of developing diabetes. Since diabetics are more susceptible to infections, this can lead to periodontitis. Periodontal disease in turn can make diabetes more difficult to control.

- Poor oral hygiene puts one at risk for kidney, pancreatic and blood cancers as well as kidney disease and possible renal failure.

- People with gum disease are four times more likely to get rheumatoid arthritis (Garrard 2016).

When patients who live with dementia benefit from the best oral hygiene possible, they will improve their quality of life and experience increased longevity. In the next chapter, I will consider how this can be achieved.

CHAPTER 2

Tips and Tricks for Optimal Oral Care

It is often very challenging to maintain good standards of oral care with people living with dementia or a mental health challenge. For this reason, it is necessary to be creative and think outside the box.

I had a patient who, for the sake of confidentiality, I will refer to as Max. He was 26 years old with a diagnosis of young onset Alzheimer's disease. Throughout his life, Max had neglected his teeth, choosing to brush them rarely and never visiting a dentist. When I met him, he had a severe case of halitosis, his teeth were badly discoloured from nicotine and coffee and it was clear there was much more gum and tooth disease that required attention.

The model I follow when implementing an intervention that requires blue sky thinking (thinking outside the box of normal, everyday clinical practice) is based on four key factors as identified in Figure 2.1.

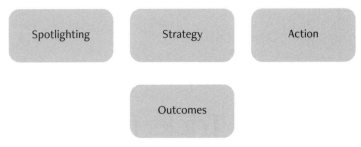

Figure 2.1: Blue sky thinking

In the case of Max, this model proved useful in achieving the aim of encouraging and supporting him to see a dentist. It is a process that any caregiver, formal or informal, can implement with equal success.

Spotlighting

This is a technique I use when I am working with a patient to identify the underlying problem that has brought them to see me. With Max, it was imperative that I uncovered why he had avoided visiting the dentist throughout his 26 years of life.

I start by establishing a therapeutic relationship, and with Max it was based around our mutual liking for music and sport, both boxing and rugby. He was very nervous, anxious and driven by fear, typical of someone living with dementia.

Once Max felt safe with me, I was able to explore the reasons for his fear of going to the dentist. As a young boy, his father had pulled one of Max's loose teeth with his fingers. It had hurt so badly he would never allow anyone to touch his teeth again.

Strategy

The next step in this model is to develop a strategy, with the patient being at the very core of any game plan created. At this stage, it was imperative that Max took the lead, made the decisions and controlled everything moving forward.

Action

Once we knew the cause of Max's anxiety around visiting the dentist, we were able to empower him in developing a strategy that put him in the driving seat of finding a resolution. It transpired that Max's favourite band was Queen, with Freddie Mercury being his rock idol. That was somewhat fortuitous because the dentist I referred him to was also a huge fan of Freddie and Queen! Together we agreed the following action:

- I would arrange for Max to go and see Dr Jones for a dental examination.

- Prior to Max's wife taking him to the dental office, she would play his favourite album, *A Kind of Magic*, both at home and in the car (it transpired that they both rocked out to this album as they made their way to see the dentist!).

- Dr Jones would play a Queen song in his office while working with Max.

Outcome

Max and his wife had an amazing surprise when they arrived at the dental office. In reception were numerous photos of Queen playing venues such as Wembley stadium. Dr Jones had also put some magazines and other memorabilia on the tables, which distracted Max from worrying about the examination, thus decreasing his anxiety levels.

Once he was in the office and in the dentist's chair, Max became engrossed in a conversation with Dr Jones about Queen. When it was time for the examination, there were no issues and a further appointment was made where Max agreed to have his teeth and gums treated.

It is essential that we think outside the box and work collaboratively to support people to live as well as possible through their unique journey of dementia.

I will now consider some tricks and tips used in the dental office that can lead to optimal oral care. These strategies require a team effort involving the patient, professionals and family members and/or friends.

TIP NUMBER 1: GETTING TO KNOW YOU

Get to know the patient – this refers to the entire dental practice team, from the receptionist to the most senior dentist.

One way of doing this is to hold a monthly 'Getting to know you. Getting to know us' event specifically aimed at families or individuals currently on their journey through cognitive change. This could be in an early evening or on a Saturday.

Provide some snacks and beverages and have all the team available. Prepare some flyers containing basic information on how the team work with people who have additional complex needs and demonstrate that every member of the team has received extra training in supporting people living with various forms of cognitive challenge.

You could also do an informal presentation and hold a Q and A session.

TIP NUMBER 2: LIFE STORY

Ensure that you have an entire history of the patient. Not only is medical information and history important, but life history too. The following page of Five things I like/Five things I don't like/ Five things I like to do/Five things I don't like to do is sufficient and can be completed with the involvement of everyone:

Five things I like	Five things I don't like
1	1
2	2
3	3
4	4
5	5
Five things I like to do	**Five things I don't like to do**
1	1
2	2
3	3
4	4
5	5

Knowing a person makes a huge difference to their sense of personhood. When referring to personhood, I include things such as sense of purpose and being, likes and dislikes, choices, individuality, personality and character. All the things that make up a person are the things that lead to personhood. The aim is always to avoid malignant social psychology, or negative care strategies, approaches and interventions that diminish an individual.

TIP NUMBER 3: POINTS OF CONVERSATION

Ensure that you have three points of conversation based on the individual's life history. I suggest the following:

1. Past or previous occupation: We spend our lives in various roles. We may be a father or mother, an auntie or uncle, a son or a daughter. We behave differently in each of these roles due to the responsibilities bestowed on us. However, one of the things that most of us hold dear and cherish is our occupation. It is often during that role that we meet people, including our future spouse, and it is where we achieve as much as we can and perform to our highest ability. Engaging in these types of conversations reminds people of their value and self-worth and has a very positive impact on their personhood.

2. Sport/leisure interest: Most people have interests outside work and this is one of the things we all cherish as part of work–life balance. Again, people often achieve things during their pursuits – being able to talk about the day Fred won the golf tournament or when Sandra won the final of the pool competition brings up fantastic memories and puts people in a really good place as far as their mental health is concerned.

3. Family (if there is no family, choose another topic such as fashion – something based on what you have

learned from the individual's life story and 'Getting to know you' event): If you ask most people, family is, and always was, their major priority throughout life. There is so much that can be discussed here, and very often, as healthcare professionals, we can relate to many of the same experiences and stories. All parents face similar experiences when bringing up children and can often speak with pride about their accomplishments. Holiday destinations and times such as Easter and Christmas are always fun to talk about.

You must be motivated to instigate the conversation and ask questions that are clear, concise and basic. We do not expect the individual to process complex information, and very often they will focus on topics and events that are based on history. *Remember:* the only time period that matters to someone living through cognitive change is the present. Whatever happened five minutes ago is irrelevant. Whatever is about to happen in five minutes' time has no impact right now. This very second, the second you are engaging with the patient, is the only action that matters. It is easy to fall into the trap of talking about upcoming events or further treatment if in the dental chair.

TIP NUMBER 4: ACTIVITIES

The reception area of a dental office can be a negative place to be. People waiting to see the dentist are often very nervous, highly anxious and afraid. These are natural feelings and emotions that most people feel when visiting a dentist or doctor of any type. Usually, there are a few magazines scattered around and perhaps a few toys for children to entertain themselves with.

Let us think about some of the day-to-day challenges faced by those experiencing their journey through dementia:

- Increased anxiety in unfamiliar surroundings

- Restlessness due to decreased ability to concentrate

- Agitation due to inability to comprehend certain experiences

- Frustration due to forgetfulness.

Challenges are likely to be unique to each individual; however, these four highlighted above are common experiences.

There are a number of ways in which we can ensure available activities in the reception area or waiting rooms that are interactive, engaging and stimulating while at the same time being age appropriate and not too challenging, or completely fail free.

First, there is adult colouring, which is a growing activity enjoyed by many throughout the world. There are some books that are relatively basic and quick to complete.

A second activity is recognition cards such as word games. For example, show a card to the person that has 'That is water under the ...' written on it and they have to find the word that completes the sentence (in this case, the word is bridge). Again, this activity is quick and can be concluded at any time.

Something that many people with neurocognitive and neurological disorders respond to is music. Playing music that the person relates to will contribute to bringing down anxiety levels and improve the person's mindset.

By talking with the person, their family and friends, and including the questions mentioned in Tip 2, the dental team will be able to identify the most appropriate activities for patients.

TIP NUMBER 5: THINK ABOUT
FLOOR AND COLOURS

Two primary colours (yellow and blue) and three secondary colours (orange, green and purple) are the best colours for dental offices and treatment rooms.

Consider that many of those living with dementia will have difficulties with their sight. This will be due to either their condition, the natural aging process or a combination of both. This further enhances feelings of confusion, disorientation and isolation. Consequently, levels of both fear and anxiety will increase.

The use of colours, especially in a contrasting way, makes a huge difference. You can highlight important areas while losing unimportant, unwanted and unneeded areas. Colour can also be used to highlight risks as well as elevate mood.

It is best to avoid the colour red as much as possible – including red clothing such as uniforms and scrubs. It is a colour that can induce rage and is often associated with danger. If we consider a red traffic sign, it means STOP.

For some people living with dementia, in particular those with Lewy Body dementia (the third leading cause of neurocognitive disorder), there is difficulty with spatial awareness. This is due to damage of the brain's posterior parietal lobe, which means awareness of oneself in space is lost. Someone with this issue struggles to understand the relationship of organized objects in a particular space when there is a positional change. People manage better on an even floor that does not change due to gradient, colour or texture. In other words, try to ensure the floor remains constant and unchanged. This can help reduce falls risk as well as improve the environment, so it is more predictable.

None of these strategies needs to be costly but all can have an extremely positive impact on the person visiting the dental office.

There are certain tricks that can be used when carrying out oral hygiene on patients who are living with cognitive or mental health challenges. I would like to point out here that these tricks are in no way intended as personal detractors (by this, I mean putting people down by disempowering them). On the contrary, these tricks are aimed at further empowering the individual to be as involved as possible with maintaining adequate levels of dental health. Here are three such strategies.

TRICK NUMBER 1: OVERCOMING SUGAR CRAVING

We are a nation of soda drinkers, and we have a great deal of information that sugar is damaging to teeth and gums and also to physical and brain health in general. We also know that sugar and refined carbs can lead to mild cognitive impairment and dementia. Therefore, my recommendation here is to replace high sugar content soda with drinks that contain natural sweetener. Of course, we should encourage people to drink plenty of water throughout the day. The trick part is changing the habit of the cue, the behaviour and the reward.

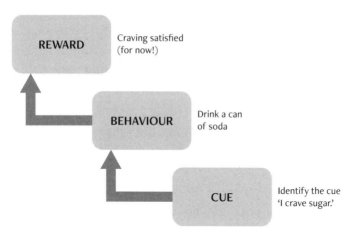

Figure 2.2: Existing habit and behaviour

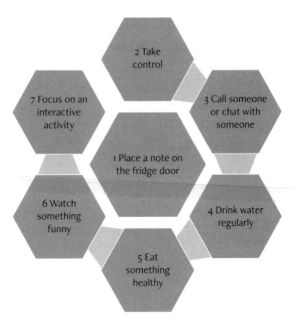

Figure 2.3: The seven actions to change the craving

1. Place a note on the fridge door that is a positive statement. For example, 'Drinking water is good for my overall health.'

2. Take control of the craving by closing your eyes, taking five deep breaths and allowing your mind to drift off to a forest or beach. This will help with relaxation and control.

3. Call someone or sit down and have a chat with a friend. This will help focus your mind on other things.

4. Ensure you drink water throughout the day. It's ok to have caffeine-free tea or coffee but ensure you have

bottled water in the fridge which you can access and drink at any time.

5. Eat something healthy – a piece of fruit would be an ideal choice!

6. Watch something funny on TV or the internet. Giving your brain a five-minute blast of funny releases a whole bunch of feel-good chemicals.

7. Focus on an interactive activity that draws your mind away from the old craving.

If this is done every day for at least two weeks, the person will be in control – and, in addition, their oral health will be improved and they may even find an improvement in cognition.

If you are a family member, friend or professional caregiver, then it will be your role to support the individual through this (it may also be a useful process for you too).

TRICK NUMBER 2: BRUSHING CAN BE FUN

It is important to brush teeth a minimum of twice daily. For those who have issues with teeth and gums, this may have to be done more frequently. We should always brush after eating, but this isn't always possible.

When supporting people who are resistant to oral hygiene or those who need assistance as part of their personal care, make the activity fun and enjoyable. Nobody is motivated when these things become a chore, so try the following to encourage better overall mouth care:

- There is a little-known happy song called *Pink Toothbrush*. You will find it on YouTube. Play it in the background – it will instil a positive mindset and make people smile! The song was released in 1959 by a guy called Max Bygraves (some of the older generation, like me, will remember him!).

- Earlier we talked about the importance of colours. Use fun-coloured toothbrushes and toothpaste tubes that contrast. Use colours that are uplifting and provide the 'feel-good' factor.

- Use as many imaginative, interactive and fun techniques that you can think of.

- It is important to empower the person to do as much for themselves as possible, but support must be provided when it is required.

TRICK NUMBER 3: DEALING WITH PAIN AND DISCOMFORT

For some people living with various types of dementia or mental health challenges, both chronic and acute pain due to infection and/or broken, decaying teeth, or teeth that are abnormal in other ways, are obvious barriers to staying on top of oral hygiene.

However, it is clearly very important that these issues are addressed and overcome in order to reduce further risks to the person's health and well-being as well as to improve overall quality of life.

First, management overseen by a dentist is the first step. Antibiotics, analgesia and other medications prescribed by a health professional must be administered as directed. Pain management is crucial, and there are various other types in addition to acute and chronic pain – for example, someone may be experiencing breakthrough pain, nerve pain or referred pain. It is essential that the right type of pain is identified so that it can be managed accordingly.

Before any oral care and intervention, ensure that the person is as pain free as possible. Administer pain relief approximately 30 minutes beforehand and also do the following relaxation technique with the individual:

1. Play some very relaxing music – *Weightless* by Marconi Union or *Watermark* by Enya are excellent examples.

2. Ask the person to close their eyes and breathe (deep breaths are best, but if this is not possible, gentle breathing will suffice). Breathe with them.

3. Once the person feels relaxed and pain free, carry out the oral hygiene process.

4. Always communicate with the person and keep them in that positive frame of mind.

CHAPTER 3

Proactive Dental and Oral Care

Over the years, we have learned a great deal about the role diet and nutrition plays in dementia. One of the most famous, and ongoing, research projects in dementia is the Nun Study. During that project, Dr David Snowdon (2001) was able to demonstrate that those nuns who had high levels of lycopene[1] had much lower incidence of dementia. In 2012, Dr Marwan Sabbagh, a US-based leading neurologist specializing in dementia, and leading chef Beau MacMillan published a book called *The Alzheimer's Prevention Cookbook,* further demonstrating the importance of certain foodstuffs as a prophylactic and proactive move towards staving off cognitive change.

There is obviously a correlation here between diet and nutrition, proactive dental and oral care and the impact the western diet has on both dementia and mental illness.

---

1   Lycopene is a red carotenoid hydrocarbon – or non-oxygen containing carotenoids – found in red fruits such as tomatoes and watermelons. Although there is no vitamin A in lycopene, it is a powerful antioxidant.

The diagram below (Figure 3.1) connects all these things together and what follows are tips for being proactive in managing dental and oral care.

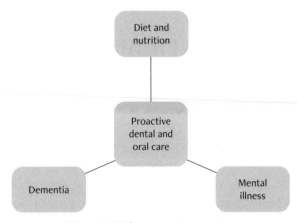

Figure 3.1: The connective strategy

So, what exactly do we mean by proactive dental and oral care in relation to those living with dementia or a mental illness? We all know we should brush our teeth at least twice a day, floss as often as possible and visit the dentist twice a year for cleaning and checks. When we are thinking rationally, are healthy and independent, then this is a straightforward habit easily developed into a routine. However, when there is cognitive change or when people are experiencing the positive symptoms of a mental illness, a different, supportive and enabling strategy needs to be in place.

In terms of diet and nutrition, according to the American Dental Association, one of the first areas to decline when one's diet is less than ideal is oral health. So, what would be a good diet? A study published in the May/June 2013 issue of *General Dentistry* (Telgi *et al.* 2013) indicated that cheese raises the pH level of saliva (normally 6.2–76) and lowers the risk of tooth decay.

On Colgate's website,[2] seven foodstuffs are identified as being healthy for teeth and gums: cheese, yogurt, leafy greens, apples, carrots, celery and almonds. There are many ways in which these foodstuffs can be incorporated into the diets of our patients, with one such way being to provide them with an information sheet containing suggestions for the types of meal they can make (an awesome salad springs to mind, where all seven foodstuffs can be included!).

Let's consider how each of these can impact positively on overall mouth, teeth and gum health.

- *Cheese* contains high levels of both phosphate and calcium. Phosphate contributes greatly to building strong teeth and bones as well as filtering waste such as urea from the kidneys. Calcium also maintains healthy teeth and gums. The protein casein strengthens tooth enamel and helps reduce the risk of cavities. If all that isn't positive enough, the majority of cheeses also taste very good! For many people with dementia, in particular those who walk a great deal throughout the day, the calorie content is also beneficial.

- *Yogurt* is another food that is high in calcium. Additionally, it has healthy bacteria such as bifidobacterium and lactobacillus which help protect gums and teeth from decay. They also serve to

2   www.colgate.com

decrease levels of hydrogen sulphide, which often leads to halitosis (bad breath). It is best to avoid yogurt that contains additives, colours and additional sugar. Encourage patients to go for natural yogurt and add their own fruit, in particular blueberries, as they are regarded as one of the superfoods for brain health.

- *Leafy greens* are many in number, all of which are healthy (preferably organic if possible). Let us consider spinach, as it is high in both calcium and folic acid, which can help in the treatment of gum disease. Beta-carotene, found in plants and fruits, especially spinach, carrots and colourful vegetables such as sweet potatoes, red and yellow peppers and apricots, is beneficial in the maintenance of strong tooth enamel. For those who fear visiting the dentist or who are not accepting of assistance with oral hygiene, encourage a daily dose of fresh spinach.

- *Apples* are well known for their benefits to teeth and gums. The acidity of an apple helps keep halitosis at bay and the apple peel contains both soluble and insoluble fibre. According to the University of Illinois, approximately two-thirds of an apple's fibre content is in its peel. Getting enough fibre in one's diet is important for maintaining a healthy digestive and cardiovascular system.

- *Carrots* are a fantastic tool for both the informal caregiver and professional healthcare worker. This is because a carrot is nature's very own toothbrush!

A daily munch on a carrot helps massage the gums, while the keratin attacks plaque. It doesn't end there either, as the vitamin A contained within this vegetable contributes to strengthening tooth enamel.

- *Celery* is high in fibre and helps clean the areas between teeth. In addition, chewing on celery helps stimulate the production of saliva, which contains bicarbonate, phosphate and our old friend calcium. These chemicals help repair damage to teeth and decay in their early stages.

- *Almonds and almond butter* have various benefits for teeth and gums. Almonds themselves can be crunched up, put on a toothbrush and used as a kind of exfoliation for teeth! This helps removes stains naturally. Almond butter has that awesome calcium as well as loads of fibre. Ensure that the almond butter used is minimally processed and contains the highest amount of fibre.

These foodstuffs can help massively with oral hygiene. Of course, teeth brushing, flossing, denture care and overall mouth cleansing are equally important.

To introduce these foodstuffs, one can be very creative. Remember the importance of cleaning teeth and taking care of the mouth between meals and fluid intake.

So, what if individuals cannot chew or otherwise eat some of the foodstuffs identified above? While the benefits will be less effective, a daily intake of supplements will help to a certain extent.

A number of published studies, including the work of Keshava Abbayya and colleagues (2015) and Yao-Tung Lee and colleagues (2017), have identified an association between periodontitis and Alzheimer's disease. Periodontitis is a gum infection that causes severe damage to the soft tissue and destroys the bone that supports the teeth. Research led by Vladimir Ilievski (2018) at the University of Illinois showed that mice with the bacteria that cause gum disease had inflammation and deterioration in their brains.

If it is known that the individual has periodontitis, then successfully treating it *may* (and there is currently no research to substantiate this statement) help slow down progression of the symptoms of dementia. The symptoms to look out for are:

- Bad breath

- Toothache

- Bright red gums

- Loose teeth

- Receding gums

- Tender gums

- Tooth loss

- Swelling or bleeding gums.

Treating periodontitis involves improved dental hygiene, professional cleaning, taking antibiotics, using antiseptics and, in some cases, medical intervention to remove unhealthy tissue with surgical procedures such as gingivectomy (removal of diseased gum tissue) and gingivoplasty (reshaping of healthy gum tissue around teeth).

Being proactive often means being responsible and visiting the dentist regularly, having regular professional cleaning and using the most appropriate toothpaste and toothbrush. Sonic toothbrushes are considered very effective in the removal of plaque due to the high vibrations they provide.

As a caregiver, family member or friend supporting someone's journey through dementia, you may have to take much of the proactive initiative to ensure adequate oral hygiene is maintained. That said, the person must always be at the centre of all care planning and care delivery and should be encouraged to be as independent as possible.

CHAPTER 4

Prioritizing Oral Care Needs

When we are supporting someone with complex medical care needs, whether physical or otherwise, we often must prioritize the meeting of those needs; and remember, it is a journey, so we are supporting family and friends too!

For this purpose, I find the following formula (Figure 4.1) useful for several reasons. First, it is inclusive; second, it is structured; third, it clarifies who has responsibility; and, finally, it empowers those on the journey to define the outcome.

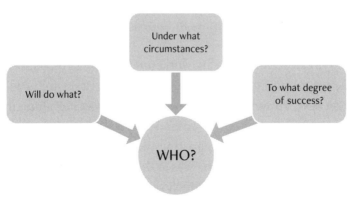

Figure 4.1: The who formula

The following case history demonstrates the usefulness of this as a tool for both formal and informal caregivers.

Helena was 68 years of age and had both amyotrophic lateral sclerosis (ALS) and frontotemporal lobar dementia (FTLD). Her needs were very complex, and she required total support to meet both Activities of Daily Living and Instrumental Activities of Daily Living (IADL). Helena was a retired, well-known and widely published archaeologist and it was difficult for her family to see the rapid decline in her physical health and changes to her behaviour, language and personality.

As she was dependent on others to meet her needs, she required 24-hour nursing and social care, which she received at the family home where she lived with her husband Cedric, and Constance, the eldest of their two daughters.

As Helena was in receipt of so much care, it was decided that a multi-disciplinary approach was required in developing a care plan that addressed her oral health, which was an area that grew increasingly challenging as her health deteriorated. The who formula was used to help achieve an effective plan and successful outcomes. Figure 4.2 demonstrates the value of using this formula in both accountability and as a structured process.

We can see that the care worker in this case had taken on the responsibility of ensuring that Helena's oral care needs were met. However, we also see that she was not alone in doing this: both family members and fellow professionals had a role to play in supporting the care worker. As must always be the case, Helena was at the centre of this element of care, being involved as much as possible.

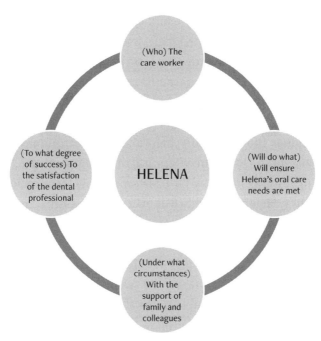

Figure 4.2: The who formula in process

The care worker, Mandy, delivered all the personal care to Helena with occasional help from both Cedric and Constance. For this reason, it was agreed that she was the best person to take the lead on oral hygiene and offer guidance and support to the rest of the multi-disciplinary team. A care plan was written that ensured both consistency and continuity of care. Two goals were set. First, Helena's teeth would be cleaned twice a day, and second, she would visit the family dentist every six months.

When Mandy was unavailable or required additional support (Helena did not always find it easy to receive personal care), family members or colleagues who made up the multi-disciplinary team, such as the community or Admiral nurse who visited daily, would lend a hand.

Dr Carlton, Helena's dentist, was the clinician responsible, and was more than prepared to see his patient whenever the need arose. He also provided Mandy with appropriate educational material and his hygienist taught her some techniques that were very helpful. These techniques were also taught to family members and other support staff.

Suggestions made by Dr Carlton and his team included changing Helena's toothbrush every four months, flossing her teeth once a day if she was comfortable with that, using a tongue scraper at least once a day and, if necessary, making use of a suction toothbrush. As Helena was no longer able to swallow, her mouth was to be swabbed twice a day with fresh pineapple juice and lemon water (this reduces the risk of xerostomia, or dry mouth).

The following is a natural mouthwash that can be used by anybody and is extremely beneficial for people living with dementia:

- Blend one cup of warm water with a quarter of a teaspoon of baking soda and an eighth of a teaspoon of pure salt (do not use table salt).

- Encourage the person to swish this around their mouth for a few seconds before rinsing out with fresh water (if the person cannot do this, use mouth swabs).

- Repeat this at three-hour intervals.

At this point, I would like readers to consider the basic nursing process of Assess, Plan, Implement and Evaluate, or APIE. We have seen how the who formula can be used as a tool for positively impacting on oral health, and now readers can learn how APIE can be used when prioritizing needs.

This process can be used by both informal caregivers and professional healthcare workers, so it is very much part of a collaborative approach to care.

Assess

Assessing the oral healthcare needs of an individual living with dementia is something the person can do themselves, a caregiver can support and a professional healthcare worker such as a dentist or dental hygienist can oversee. In previous chapters, we have learned about the essential aspects of oral hygiene and its maintenance, but what other priorities are there when meeting the psychological and physiological needs of people living with the challenges of dementia or mental illness? The answer to this is dependent on the individual and where in their journey they are at the time of assessment (and remember the phrase 'each day different, every day new' when supporting people through their journey).

Let us consider Alison, a 59-year-old lady with a diagnosis of Lewy Body dementia. We need to consider her overall care needs and determine their priorities.

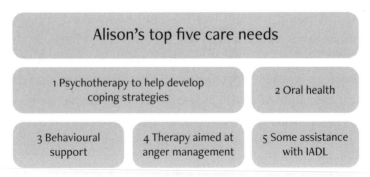

Figure 4.3. Alison's top five care needs

Following assessment by the Admiral nurse leading Alison's dementia care, five top priorities were identified (see Figure 4.3). Alison's husband and two daughters were part of the assessment process.

The diagnosis was recent (delivered only a few weeks earlier) so everyone felt that she desperately needed to develop some coping strategies to deal with the challenges she and her family faced at the present time and as her unique journey progressed. However, up until the past six months, Alison had always prided herself on her appearance and met her oral hygiene needs without any difficulty. The lack of interest in that aspect was raised as a concern by the family, thus making that part of her care priority number 2.

Plan

For the purpose of this chapter, I am going to focus solely on the plan for meeting Alison's oral hygiene needs.

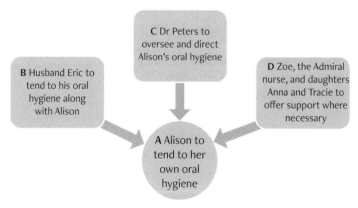

Figure 4.4: Plan of action

A Alison had the physical ability to carry out the directions provided by Dr Peters in order to meet her own oral hygiene needs. However, as she travelled further along the journey of Lewy Body dementia, this would change. Therefore, it was decided that they would all be proactive and put strategies in place so that Alison would get used to them over time. The aim here was to make the transition from independence to supported care and intervention a smooth one.

B Eric would join Alison when it was time for brushing teeth, rinsing with mouthwash and flossing. He would also attend dental appointments at the same time as his wife. Once this behaviour became routine and habitual, it was less likely to be abandoned and more likely to remain familiar during the process of cognitive change. In addition, Alison would be more accepting of Eric's input.

C Having guidance and direction from the dentist was crucial, as was visiting a dentist who understood the challenges faced by Alison and her family. Dr Peters had been their family dentist for many years, so already had a trusting relationship with them all. He took the time to study how best to support a patient with dementia and felt able to continue providing general dental care.

D Having the additional support of Zoe, Anna and Tracie when needed provided assurance to both Alison and Eric, and they too learned about supporting the oral hygiene of someone living with this type of dementia.

Implement

It was decided that, for now, Alison would be encouraged to brush and floss twice a day and reminded that it might be a good idea to have a quick brush after taking medication or eating. She had used a sonic toothbrush for several years and agreed to continue using it. As her journey moved forward, the family agreed to review this plan.

Evaluate

As with any plan, its impact must be evaluated. As clinical lead, Zoe discussed this with the family, who all agreed that monthly reviews and evaluations would take place. However, if things changed between times this would be brought forward.

Tips for meeting oral hygiene needs

A Lewy Body dementia organization in Canada,[1] which provides information on learning to live with this type of dementia, offers the following tips for everyone when meeting oral hygiene needs:

- Make a routine, and a safe place to do it, where the person is comfortable and confident. At a table with a basin or at the sink with a chair may be best.

- Provide a mirror so that they can recognize what they're doing – a movable or portable one may be better than a fixed one, to allow different positions.

- Try a power toothbrush on a low setting – this can be very efficient and will reduce the need for back-and-forth movement, which can be difficult, frustrating and unpleasant. If the sensation of the power toothbrush makes the person uncomfortable, discontinue it at least temporarily, or use the power only for very difficult-to-reach areas.

- Consider using a child's toothbrush, which is smaller, may be easier to manipulate in a confined space and has softer bristles that may reduce unpleasant sensations.

---

1   http://lewybodydementia.ca

- Remember that toothpaste may be counterproductive and unnecessary if its taste, frothiness, volume and spitting-out requirements pose problems. Organic or children's toothpaste has fewer potential issues if accidentally swallowed, and a gel form may be preferable to the grittier texture of some toothpastes.

- If possible, dilute the toothpaste to make a thinner consistency to eliminate any blobs that could potentially mix with saliva and increase the risk of choking.

- If flossing is very difficult, try things like Plackers floss picks, Stimudents and Water-Pik devices to make this easier.

- Ensure that they spit out as much as possible when finished to avoid potential swallowing issues or stomach upset.

- Be careful to avoid choking, aspiration and respiratory impacts by careful attention to posture, fatigue, attention and distractions.

- Remember that some medications can be very damaging to teeth and gums, so whenever possible, do a light brushing or mouth rinse after taking medications, especially if they are taken crushed in food.

- If necessary, take more frequent trips to the dentist for professional cleaning, especially if frequent brushing and cleaning is difficult to accomplish.

Early stage unassisted brushing tips

- Encourage and facilitate oral hygiene as effectively as possible to minimize future problems and to maintain habit and comfort level.

- Make sure that the location used for toothbrushing is safe; this could mean providing a chair at the sink or a portable basin and brush at the table the person eats at.

- Keep the implements rigorously clean, close at hand, with easy-to-grip handles and contrasting colours so they're easy to see and use if hand–eye coordination diminishes.

- Periodically check up on the efficiency of brushing and flossing in case it is not being done but you assume it is.

- If self-directed brushing and flossing are not being done well, you can facilitate this and improve the results significantly by brushing your own teeth at the same time as the person. 'Mirroring' is commonly used and is simply doing the desired behaviour yourself so the person doesn't have to remember, they can just see what you are doing and imitate the desired activity.

- Do your own teeth at the same time, in clear view of the person, so they can mimic what you're doing closely.

- Maintain a pleasant aspect and avoid annoyance or scolding. Encourage positively: the person may be unclear on what's needed, so use very clear, simple instructions if helpful.

- Make sure there's time after every meal to brush, because the person may be too tired otherwise, and particles of food left in the mouth can cause many serious problems.

- Use an egg-timer or non-disconcerting alarm to make sure the brushing goes on long enough to be thorough.

Advanced stage assistance and brushing someone's teeth

If a person is too tired, confused or unable to do the brushing themselves, you will need to help them partially, or do it yourself. With ingenuity, patience and care, this can be easy to do in many cases. It brings great benefits for hygiene and drastically diminishes the likelihood of aspiration and pneumonia (from food particles dislodging and ending up in the lungs).

- Brush your own teeth just before helping them with theirs to visually establish what's expected and appropriate, and so they know that it is not something being done 'to' them, but 'for' them.

- Get all the implements you will need and keep them in sight before you start: toothbrush, towel, wash cloth, water cup, basin and so on. If they see these in advance, it should be less worrisome when you start. And seeing that the brush just went in the water in a glass or under a tap will provide assurance that it's clean.

- Describe each individual step before you do it, and show them what you mean, such as, 'I'm going to brush your teeth now, and this is the brush I will use. I'm going to put it to your lips. When you open your mouth, I'll be very gentle and clean your teeth.' Reassure them and gently explain each step before you perform it, using the simplest language possible. Singing, humming or playing soft music may help.

- Use an apron, bib or towel draped over a wide area beneath their chin to catch any drops or spit. Be extra gentle. Their gums may be very sensitive. Use the smallest, softest brush you can find.

- Ensure that your actions do not make them think you might obstruct their breathing.

- Be patient and comforting, and extra sensitive to how they react. Having an unpleasant experience with brushing can elicit difficult behaviour and reduce your status as a person they trust intuitively.

- If it is creating agitation, stop for a while.

- Play quiet, favoured, calming music before and during to help reduce agitation. Avoid other seen, heard or felt distractions while brushing.

- Make it a ritual. Be as consistent with the process as possible. Keeping the routine the same all the time will allow whatever memory abilities remain to help you by making it less upsetting by its familiarity. Even if they never become calm, once you establish your own routine, you will be calmer yourself, and that will lead to less potential agitation or anxiety.

- Support the person at eye level, make physical contact, remain in their field of vision and avoid threatening postures or gestures.

We often use the term 'It takes a village to care for a person.' When it comes to supporting someone through their journey of dementia, a collaborative team approach is the only way to ensure improved quality of life. Our aim is always to help people maintain as much control over decision making and to remain as independent as possible. This is how we achieve personhood, and the more we learn about cognitive change and how to slow down or arrest its progress, the more we are able to help people living with dementia.

We have the same view about mental illness and the many challenges it brings to those living with it. APIE is also a valuable process when supporting those with active psychoses as well as those living with neurotic disorders such as chronic anxiety, phobias, clinical depression and obsessive-compulsive disorders. These can have a major impact on oral hygiene and need to be addressed.

The fear of toothbrushes (odontoarruphobia) needs to be treated through psychotherapy, hypnotherapy or/ and cognitive behaviour therapy. The same can be said of obsessive-compulsive disorders, depression and anxiety. It is also worth bearing in mind that psychosis, neurosis and dementia can co-exist, therefore bringing even further challenges to the individual, family and healthcare professionals.

Education about the importance of oral hygiene is essential, and I suggest that adequate training be provided to families and those working in the care home and domiciliary care services. This area of care must always be seen as a top priority, with the dentists and their staff viewed as an integral part of any multi-disciplinary team approach to care.

CHAPTER 5

How to Spot Oral Disease and Action Interventions

How does someone living with dementia or active mental health challenges, their family members, formal caregivers and professional oral health practitioners identify disease of the teeth, gums and mouth?

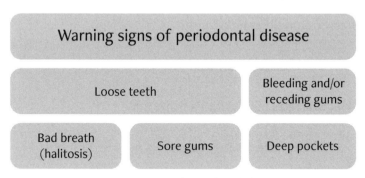

Figure 5.1: Signs of periodontal disease

Periodontitis is a serious gum infection that, if left untreated, can destroy the jawbone. Clearly, prevention is better than treatment, but being able to recognize the warning signs offers the best clinical outcomes to treatment.

Figure 5.1 identifies the signs to look out for. If any of them are spotted, access professional dental treatment immediately.

Periodontitis affects gums before teeth, therefore, intervening as soon as gums begin to bleed or recede is crucial. If not, the infection may damage gum tissue and bone. If teeth have been affected, a technique called periodontal splinting may help. This is where weak teeth are splinted together, which turns them into a single unit. They will then be stable and much stronger. However, the aim is to avoid treatment through early intervention.

Bad breath, or halitosis, when caused by oral problems usually smells like rotten eggs. The odour is caused by the breakdown of an amino acid called cysteine. If someone suddenly develops bad breath (which can occasionally smell like faeces), and you know it isn't due to something they have eaten, seek dental help without delay. There are other causes that result in different odours:

- Nasal disease may lead to a cheesy odour.

- Diabetes may lead to a fruity odour.

- Kidney disease may produce a fishy or ammonia odour.

- Those with asthma or cystic fibrosis may have breath that smells acidic.

- Cirrhosis of the liver often produces a sweet, musty odour.

- If someone has a bowel obstruction there may be a faecal odour.

There are 12 different types of breath odour, each caused by different diseases. People living with dementia or various mental illness may experience any one of these diseases, so remain vigilant and seek medical or dental help if you notice any of them. They are:

- Diabetes breath

- Menstrual breath

- Sinus breath

- Drug breath

- Drug-induced bad breath

- Lung breath

- Halitophobia (the fear of having bad breath!)

- Tonsil breath

- Gut breath

- Trimethylaminuria breath (inability to break down this pungent odorous chemical that smells like urine, garbage or rotting fish)

- Liver breath

- Metabolic breath.

Tender, red or swollen gums are one of the reasons people may avoid cleaning their teeth. If this is the case, encourage them to rinse their mouth with a saltwater solution to help remove any bacteria lurking inside the mouth. Things such as strong mouthwashes should be avoided, and alcohol should be replaced with plenty of water. Gum pain can also be lessened by supporting the person to place a warm compress over their face (this might not be something you or your relative/friend can tolerate, but it is worth a try as it is very effective). Another leading cause of swollen gums is the very common and contagious virus herpes simplex labialis (cold sores), particularly if it is recurrent. This should be treated with antiviral medicines. It is important to have the input of the dentist or GP to help with long-term management. However, use of a cold compress can help reduce any swelling or inflammation.

Deep (or periodontal) pockets can lead to tooth loss. According to Colgate, if your mouth is healthy, gums should fit snugly around the teeth with a distance between gum tissue and the attachment to the tooth being only a few millimetres in depth. If pockets become deep, with early diagnosis and treatment this can be managed. Scaling and root planing by the dental team will remove all the tartar and plaque, which will help the gums heal and once again tighten around the teeth.

In addition to managing oral hygiene, your dentist can detect other diseases such as diabetes, leukaemia, oral and pancreatic cancer as well as heart and kidney disease.

Baby boomers (those born between 1946 and 1964) are especially vulnerable to developing diabetes, osteoporosis and heart disease, the risks of which increase with age. Researchers believe that symptoms of these conditions can manifest in the mouth, making dentists key in diagnosing the diseases. For example:

- Bad breath and bleeding gums could be indicators of diabetes

- Dental x-rays can show the first stages of bone loss

- A sore and painful jaw could foreshadow an oncoming heart attack.

Sometimes, people have difficulty feeling or expressing pain. There are cases from clinical practice where people have fallen and fractured the neck of the femur (broken hip – a very painful injury) but several days have passed before it is diagnosed. Very often, this is due to difficulty in being able to tell someone there is something wrong.

Additionally, people may be taking analgesia to manage existing, targeted pain from conditions such as arthritis, thus masking dental problems.

There are some signs you can observe that may indicate someone is in additional pain (see Figure 5.2).

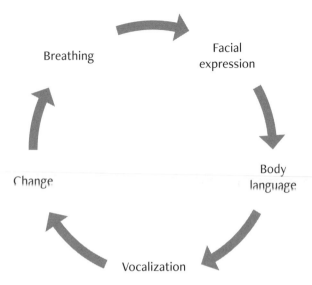

Figure 5.2: The five signs of pain and discomfort

- *Breathing* – Is breathing normal or is it laboured with periods of hyperventilation? Normal breathing is a positive sign, but if the person's breathing is different from usual and short bursts of hyperventilation are present, it may be indicative that pain is present.

- *Facial expression* – Does the person smile the majority of the time? If so, that's positive. There may be discomfort if the person looks sad, frowns a great deal, grimaces or looks frightened.

- *Body language* – Is the person relaxed and calm? Of course, this is a good sign. However, if they are fidgeting, pacing or seeming tense, check for pain.

- *Vocalization* – If there is occasional moaning or repeated calling out, groaning or crying, investigate for pain.

- *Change* – Has the person's behaviour changed for reasons you cannot see? Does comforting the person fail to assure or alleviate any unwanted behaviour? If so, this could also be indicative of pain.

There are now a number of mobile dental companies and it is recommended that this service be used for people who are further along their journey of dementia.

CHAPTER 6

Oral Care and Mental Health

People living with any kind of challenge to their mental health and well-being are likely to face issues with oral healthcare. An article published in the *Nepal Journal of Epidemiology* by Swati Gupta and colleagues (2016) states that mental illness such as schizophrenia may cause deterioration in oral health by affecting the person's ability to perform oral hygiene measures.

If we were to couple a form of mental illness such as schizophrenia, schizoaffective disorder or bipolar disorder with a neurocognitive disorder such as Alzheimer's disease, the challenge to the individual's physical and psychological health and well-being becomes even more problematic for everyone supporting that journey.

Currently in the UK, there is conflicting information regarding the availability and quality of dental treatment and oral care, with many dentists making comparisons with third-world countries and NHS England counter-arguing that things are improving. In a 2018 letter to *The Daily Telegraph* (Evans 2018), dentists made the point that oral health in Britain was becoming a national disgrace and a national health disaster. The Oral Health Foundation argues that anxiety and panic attacks, depression, eating disorders, obsessive-compulsive disorder and self-harm, in addition to schizophrenia and psychosis(es), also have a negative impact on an individual's oral health. It states that those living with a mental illness tend to avoid dental care so much that their oral hygiene is neglected, thus resulting in both gum disease and tooth decay. Medication taken to help manage both psychosis(es) and neurosis(es) may also have an impact, including dry mouth (xerostomia) due to reduced flow of saliva.

By applying the following interactional enablement model, those supporting the individual through their unique and complex journey can positively influence high standards of oral hygiene and dental care. I have demonstrated how this model can be used through a real-life case study within my own practice as a clinical dementia specialist (names changed to adhere to patient confidentiality and preserve the anonymity of professionals and family members involved).

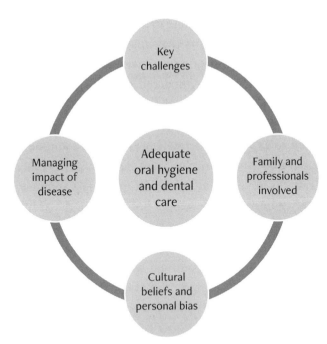

Figure 6.1: Interactional enablement model

Francine was a 52-year-old lady with a recent diagnosis of young onset Alzheimer's disease. For approximately five years she had been treated for severe anxiety disorder and clinical depression. Since the age of 17, Francine had also lived with paranoid schizophrenia. This multi-pathology of disease meant that her care plan would be very complex and require multi-disciplinary input. It became evident at our very first consultation that she had halitosis and discoloured teeth. I noted that this would need to be included in any treatment plan I proposed, with Francine being enabled to make decisions about her entire care plan.

If we consider the above interactional enablement model that was used with Francine, we see that at the very core is our key, long-term goal: adequate oral hygiene and dental care. We identified four factors that needed to be addressed in order to achieve that goal. First, it was essential to pin down the key challenges that impacted on Francine's everyday life. Second, we needed to establish which professionals and family members would be involved in her journey. Third, I needed to explore Francine's cultural beliefs and her own personal bias (including her own belief system regarding her complex physical and mental health illness and disease). Finally, we needed to develop a holistic shared action plan that would serve to minimize the impact that living with young onset Alzheimer's disease, severe anxiety disorder, clinical depression and paranoid schizophrenia had on her life. It was evident that symptomatic management was the major challenge of everyone involved with the care of this lady. Let us now examine how we achieved our goal with Francine.

Defining adequate oral hygiene and dental care

For Francine, visiting a dentist had never been a priority. We discussed how gum disease and tooth decay impact on so many aspects of life, as well as physical health such as heart disease. She had very low self-esteem and did not take any pride in her appearance or personal hygiene. However, she eventually agreed that she would like to work on her appearance, which included visiting a dentist for the first time in over nine years. My role was to help improve her self-esteem and self-worth. In terms of defining adequate oral hygiene and dental care for Francine, we both agreed on the following statement: *'I will visit the dentist for a check-up and cleaning. I will follow the advice and guidance of the dentist and I will brush twice daily – in addition to brushing after I have taken my medication.'* That was a great start to the shared action plan.

When this is done with a family member or patient, it may take some time to explore various reasons for not visiting a dentist or brushing one's teeth. The secret is to put the individual in charge – to empower them to make decisions – while providing information, guidance and support.

Key challenges

It is crucial to identify the daily challenges faced by the individual. In this case, it was essential to define clearly the obstacles that Francine experienced in terms of basic activities of daily living and instrumental activities of daily living. Remember, she had severe anxiety disorder and clinical depression in addition to cognitive decline and schizophrenia, therefore motivation and drive needed to be a focal point. She had no physical issues with meeting personal hygiene needs, tidying the house, visiting the dentist or meeting all her other needs independently. Francine's main obstacle to overcome was her belief that there was no point in doing any of these things. We made a list of all the reasons for getting up in the morning and put together a daily schedule, which placed great emphasis on two minutes of teeth brushing in the morning, taking a shower and dressing for the day. Francine found this structured approach to be useful. The schedule was placed in an area of the house where she would see it regularly, thus helping to jog her memory. When it came to her mental illness, she experienced command (auditory), visual and gustatory (taste) hallucinations (this will be discussed in the part of the model that deals with managing the impact of the disease).

When doing this with a family member or patient, it is crucial to focus on the individual's existing strengths, competencies, abilities and interests. Regular teeth cleaning is imperative, and if the person is taking any kind of medication on a daily basis, encouraging them to brush immediately afterwards, and prior to going to bed, can make a huge difference.

Family and professionals involved

In the case of Francine, her sister was her only close and involved relative. They were supported by the psychiatrist, community mental health nurse, me as clinical dementia specialist and my preferred dentist (many of her patients had enduring mental illness and she had previously been a registered mental health nurse).

A multi-disciplinary team approach with the person at the core is essential for achieving optimal healthcare and set goals. Each professional and family member involved has a particular role, and regular communication between everyone is extremely important. When working with a dentist, it is important to find someone who is experienced at working with people who have a mental illness.

Cultural beliefs and personal bias

Cultural influence and personal bias play a part in developing one's mindset around oral hygiene, regardless of one's health status. For example, those raised in low-income families, those with special needs and those raised in rural areas have greater risks of oral disease. This was the case with Francine. She was never encouraged to brush her teeth or visit the dentist by her parents and rarely attended appointments with the school dentist. Other childhood experiences (not relevant here) were factors that led to Francine's severe anxiety disorder and clinical depression. Basically, we tend to live our lives via the ABC principle. The **A**ctivating event is something that triggers our response. Our response is based on our **B**elief system, which determines our response, and the **C**onsequences of our actions result from our **B**elief system. In the case of Francine, the activating event related to her parents seeing oral hygiene and dental care as unimportant. She went on to develop this belief system and as a consequence she ended up, through neglect, developing gum disease and tooth decay.

Through the interactional enablement model, we can address and change cultural beliefs, personal bias and negative attitudes towards oral health with our family members and patients.

Managing impact of disease

As we identified earlier, Francine had multi-pathology that required a very complex medical treatment plan with active therapy. Paranoid schizophrenia affected her quality of life mainly because of command, gustatory and visual hallucinations. Without appropriate medication and psychotherapy, this would be unbearable for her. The command hallucinations often instructed her to do things like place a shoe in the toilet bowl and smear jam on a window. Fortunately, they were never a risk to herself or others. The gustatory hallucinations led her to tasting something that wasn't present. This was very mild, and she experienced this kind of hallucination irregularly. It was the visual hallucinations that affected Francine in a more serious way. They were more frequent and were often things that appeared directly in front of her. They were sometimes people, other times animals or unfamiliar and unrecognizable objects. Fortunately, her psychiatrist and mental health nurse had her paranoid schizophrenia very well managed, along with the clinical depression and severe anxiety disorder. However, I decided to introduce weekly psychotherapy to support the management programme. I treated the behavioural and psychological symptoms of dementia through psychotherapy and cognitive behaviour therapy, and Francine's sister, Erica, who lived in the same town and only a few streets away, took responsibility for the following:

- Ensuring Francine took her medications on time and brushed her teeth afterwards.

- Accompanying her sister to dental appointments (these were weekly for the first four weeks until the dentist got on top of the gum disease and tooth decay).

- Assisting her to follow the daily schedule we put in place, which included oral hygiene.

- Completing any homework given as part of therapy.

- Acting as liaison between all professionals.

Family members are part of the multi-disciplinary team. They are part of the journey and have a very valuable role to play. When it comes to teeth cleaning, attending dental appointments and following the dentist's instructions, closely involved family members are our backbone. Without them (and sometimes there are no family members or close friends) our role as professionals is far more difficult.

The outcome we set out to achieve was met over a period of six months. Francine's mental illnesses was well managed, as was her young onset Alzheimer's disease. A number of teeth were extracted and replaced, the gum disease was managed effectively, and Francine's quality of life improved as a result.

This model can be used by anyone and is a structured way in which to meet any set goals.

CHAPTER 7

The Positive Dental Experience

Ask yourself this question: 'Do I relish and look forward to my dental appointment?' If you answered no, you are in the majority. If you answered yes, you are a minority (or the dentist!). However, it is likely that your body experiences a number of physiological and psychological changes as you get closer to the dentist's office.

In my book, *A Clinician's Guide to Non-Pharmacological Dementia Therapies*, (2019), Chapter 5 focuses on something called the Nightingale Dementia Triangle (Figure 7.1). It discusses how fear and anxiety play a massive role in producing the behavioural and psychological symptoms of dementia.

What we see prior to any intervention based on positive engagement is that dementia is the central actor, supported in its role by anxiety and fear. These fuel the symptoms we see in those living with cognitive decline, leading to an ever-diminishing individual.

This triangle is a very useful tool to use prior to a person living with dementia visiting the dentist, during the visit and afterwards. The aim is to change how anxiety and fear impact on the individual during these events (Figure 7.2). It can be used by the person themselves and everyone supporting their journey, including family members, the dental team and any other involved professionals.

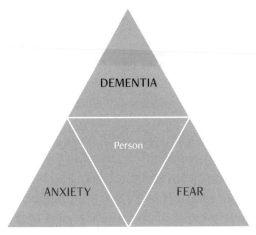

Figure 7.1: The Nightingale Dementia Triangle (pre-intervention)

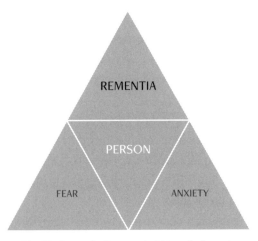

Figure 7.2: The Nightingale Dementia Triangle (post-intervention)

In order to achieve the state of well-being we are seeing in the second triangle, where the dementia symptoms have been reversed (the word we use for this is rementia, a term coined by the late Professor Tom Kitwood in 1996 to describe how individuals experiencing cognitive change can show improvement in functioning), we must address the following:

1. Choosing the right dentist – some dentists have completed additional training in order to work with people who have Alzheimer's disease or other forms of dementia. If you can find such trained professionals, they would be the ones to work with.

2. Empowering the individual to be in control of (a) making the appointment and (b) attending the appointment. The appointment should take place during a part of the day when the person functions best. Always avoid the time where people may experience sundowning (this is a neurological phenomenon associated with increased confusion and restlessness in some people living with dementia).

3. Supporting the person in bringing down their levels of both fear and anxiety about going to visit the dentist (try to arrange a visit the day prior to the actual appointment, preferably after the dentist closes their office for the day. This will help orientate the person and familiarize them with the layout and the staff team). Don't be concerned

about the person forgetting, as the most important time to a person living with cognitive change is the present. Record the layout and do a short interview with the dentist (or whoever will be carrying out the procedures). This can be viewed regularly by the individual prior to attending the appointment. On the morning of the appointment, before leaving the house, share the video with the individual; also, prior to entering the dentist's building.

4. Ensuring that you take along an engaging, interactive activity to occupy the individual while in the waiting room. Some dental offices have become 'dementia friendly' in terms of environment and staff training, and this will make the event much more straightforward, but it's a good idea to be prepared for experiences that are not like this.

5. Being present with the individual all the time. Whether we are living with dementia or not, we have the same thing in common – increased anxiety when visiting the dentist! Think about this for a moment: people living with dementia may lose control over many aspects of their lives. It is very common for people to feel helpless and a further loss of control when in the dentist's chair. If you are supporting someone in this situation, it would be helpful to come up with a strategy that empowers as opposed to disempowers them. A great way to do this is to encourage the dentist to explain everything they are doing throughout the entire procedure.

Rule number one when supporting people through their unique journey is to strive to reduce fear and anxiety. If this can be achieved in relation to visiting the dental team, there should be reduced challenges in meeting the individual's need for adequate oral hygiene and dental care.

CHAPTER 8

Interactive Case Studies

Case study 1: Harold Moon

Harold is a 78-year-old gentleman living at home with his wife Sally. Three times a week, a caregiver provides three hours of support to Harold. He wears full dentures and has had a long history of gum disease. For the past 12 months, Harold has been living with both Alzheimer's disease and prostate cancer. More recently, he has undergone a heart valve repair. The advice he and Sally have been given is that his dentures must be kept clean, his gum disease managed and his mouth kept free of bacteria.

Think about developing a care plan that Sally can use with her husband in order to help achieve adequate oral hygiene.

Suggested shared action plan for Harold

This shared action plan is intended to empower Harold to be the central driver of his own oral hygiene.

Sally and the caregiver take responsibility for supporting, enabling and empowering Harold to do as much as possible himself. Maintaining independence and dignity is crucial.

Recording a short video for Harold to follow (a form of mirroring) is aimed at maintaining independence, while reminding him to clean his dentures after every meal will reduce the risk of bacteria build-up that could lead to aspiration pneumonia.

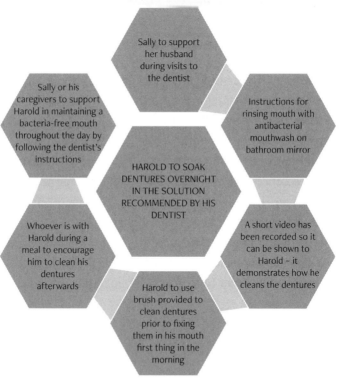

Figure 8.1: Harold's shared action plan

Case study 2: Colin Hindle

Colin is 54 years of age with a diagnosis of young onset dementia. In addition, he has Down's syndrome and a mild learning disability. He lives in a group home with five others and has always been resistant to support with oral hygiene. As a consequence, a number of his teeth have been extracted and he refuses to put a toothbrush in his mouth.

Think about developing a care plan that can be used by the care team to help achieve adequate oral hygiene.

Suggested shared action plan for Colin

Supporting Colin will bring many challenges due to the complexity of his pre-existing learning disability and Down's syndrome as well as living with young onset dementia.

In order to enable him to maintain as much independence as possible, it is necessary to establish Colin's existing strengths, abilities, likes and dislikes. Tangible rewards and outcomes must also be identified. Then, the main challenges can be prioritized and addressed through the most appropriate intervention.

Colin likes rock music; he enjoys singing; he likes to watch films and his favourite treat is playing Uno. He also enjoys a bottle of beer.

The five key challenges are identified in Figure 8.2, and the table below that considers each challenge, provides a suggested action and the desired outcome.

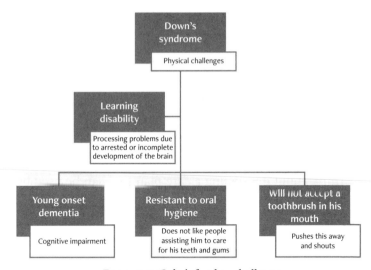

Figure 8.2: Colin's five key challenges

Table 8.1: Colin's action plan in detail

CHALLENGE	SUGGESTED ACTION	DESIRED OUTCOME
Colin has a number of physical challenges due to Down's syndrome. The one we are focusing on here is congenital heart disease. He tires very easily and also has some breathing difficulties.	Ensure that there is a chair in the bathroom and play his favourite music. Sing along with Colin to help create a positive mindset.	Colin will be relaxed and much more open to being assisted and supported during the process of oral hygiene.

Due to having a learning disability, Colin finds it difficult to process what is being asked of him.	Mirror what you want him to do. Explain everything you are doing and ensure that you add an element of fun to it.	Colin will follow your actions – especially if it is fun.
Colin's cognitive change in the form of young onset dementia affects his short-term memory. Therefore, constant reminders and prompts are essential.	Reward Colin with a game of Uno immediately on his completion of cleaning his teeth (see below for the best way to do this).	Colin will clean his teeth by mirroring the caregiver in anticipation of positive engagement through playing Uno.
A resistance to allowing anyone to support him while cleaning his teeth, gums and mouth has led to a number of lost teeth, bad breath and ongoing tooth decay.	Agree with Colin that he will let you help him twice a day. Once you have done this, you can either watch a film together, play Uno or have a beer.	Colin's oral hygiene will improve. As he grows more used to a consistent approach in teeth cleaning, he will become more relaxed and less resistant.
Throughout his entire life, Colin has resisted having a toothbrush in his mouth. There could be a number of reasons for this, but that is not important. The important element is that he be encouraged to overcome this issue through empowerment.	Accompany Colin to the shop so he can choose a toothbrush (preferably a sonic one that he likes). Then, give lots of encouragement through mirroring (personally or via a video) with an immediate reward. Encourage Colin to do it for himself.	By mirroring you or following a fun video (something you may wish to make yourself), Colin will be in control of the brush. The immediate reward (and reminder that there is a reward) will help achieve the desired outcome of improved oral hygiene.

These are just some suggestions. The only right way is the one that works for the individual.

Case study 3: Molly Saunders

Molly is 83 years old, lives in a care home for nursing care and has a mild cognitive impairment. She has severe arthritis throughout the majority of her body and requires support in meeting all her basic activities of daily living. When it comes to assistance with personal care, Molly is very resistant and the staff team find it a real challenge to maintain oral hygiene. Molly still has some of her teeth remaining, though many of them have been extracted.

Think about developing a care plan with Molly that can be used by the care team to help achieve adequate oral hygiene.

Suggested shared action plan for Molly

Molly has a great personality and sense of humour. She is very friendly and kind and is a great story teller. She has a mild cognitive impairment and is resistant to personal care. When it comes to oral hygiene, she tends to be very resistant though will say things like, 'I only have seven teeth. No point cleaning them!'

The following is a suggested approach and intervention.

1. Molly enjoys engaging in banter with her care team.

2. She has much respect for her GP (who has been a family friend since he was a child) and always does as he asks.

3. Molly has enough awareness that keeping her mouth free of bacteria, her gums as clean as possible and the seven remaining teeth healthy are all important for her physical well-being.

Actions:

- Engage Molly in as much 'fun' discussion as possible – also, share with her clips from comedy shows which she enjoys (especially her favourite – *The Two Ronnies!*).

- Ask the GP to record a short, two-minute video on Molly's phone reinforcing the importance of cleaning her teeth and maintaining healthy mouth and gums.

- Reward Molly with something of her choice once she has permitted you to help with oral care.

Remember, empowering Molly to be proactive and independent in her own oral hygiene will lead to a much more positive outcome.

CHAPTER 9

General Questions and Answers

Following discussion with care partners of people living with dementia at various stages, the following top five questions and answers have been compiled.

Question 1

Is there any medication that people with dementia take that impacts on oral hygiene?

Every time medication is taken, the person should brush their teeth as part of an ongoing habit. The more it becomes routine, the less challenging it will be. Through a process called repetitive muscular activity (which means repeating the same movements and motions over and over again) it is possible for the brain to lay down new neural pathways. This is a way in which the brain can learn a new skill or relearn a lost one. In dementia terms, we refer to this as rementia (an improvement in function).

People with dementia are sometimes prescribed antidepressants, antipsychotics and sedatives. One of the side effects of all these drugs is a dry mouth. Saliva acts as a lubricant, and dry mouth can cause problems with dentures, including discomfort and looseness. Denture fixatives and artificial saliva can help some people with denture problems. Once again, the dentist can provide advice.

Saliva not only acts as a lubricant, but also has a cleansing effect on the mouth and teeth. Its absence leads to plaque accumulation, gum disease and dental decay, particularly at the neck of the tooth. Decay in this area undermines the crown of the tooth and can cause the crown to break off.

If medication is syrup-based, there is an increased danger of tooth decay. Your doctor may be able to prescribe a sugar-free alternative if asked. The dentist may also be able to apply chlorhexidine and fluoride varnishes to help prevent decay at the necks of the teeth. Reduction of sugar in the diet, particularly sugary snacks, also helps to control decay. Some antipsychotic drugs can cause increased tongue and jaw movements, making it difficult to wear dentures, particularly in the lower jaw. Unfortunately, these jaw tremors may remain after the drug is stopped.

The following list gives families of medications that can lead to tooth decay and other oral problems:

- Antihistamines

- Decongestants

- Antihypertensives, used to treat hypertension (high blood pressure), including diuretics

- Antidepressants

- Sedatives

- Analgesics

- Antacids, used to neutralize stomach acidity, relieving heartburn, indigestion and an upset stomach

- Levodopa, used in conjunction with carbidopa to treat the symptoms of Parkinson's disease such as shakiness and difficulty moving.

If any of these medications are being taken, it is crucial that extra oral hygiene care is implemented.

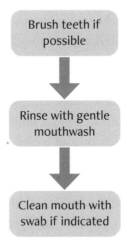

Figure 9.1: Procedure to follow after taking medicine

The first option is to brush the teeth for at least two minutes after taking medication. Before doing so, ensure all the medicine has been swallowed.

The person can also rinse the mouth with a gentle antiseptic mouthwash – if it is not possible to brush the teeth then try to get the person to do this.

If it is not possible to brush the teeth or rinse the mouth, for example if someone is receiving end-of-life care, then it may be necessary to clean the mouth with dental swabs.

Whatever the scenario, it is essential to be extra vigilant if people are taking medication.

Always follow the instructions provided by the dentist or other healthcare professional as each individual is unique.

Question 2

How do I access a dentist who is trained to work with people living with dementia? What questions should I ask?

If you are seeking a new dentist, it is essential to find a dental practice where staff have had additional training to work with people living with dementia and those experiencing active challenges to their mental health.

There are training programmes available for dental teams, though not all enrol on them. Inner-city dentists are more likely to have more patients living with dementia or an active mental illness on their list than rural practices.

It might be a good idea to check with the Alzheimer's Society, or other voluntary organizations, to ask if they are aware of any dentists in your local area who may have had additional training.

Here are some questions you should ask when finding the right dental practice:

- Have you and your team had additional training in supporting people who have dementia or an active mental health challenge?

- Are any team members Dementia Friends?

- Are you happy to work with my husband/wife etc. Explain clearly what challenges the individual is experiencing, especially in relation to basic activities and instrumental activities of daily living.

- Do you have additional time or are your appointments time sensitive?

- Take into consideration the environment – is the lighting adequate? Are the colours appropriate? Is the flooring appropriate? Refer to Chapter 7 when considering the environment of the dental practice.

Question 3

How do I assess my family member's oral hygiene status?

If you or your family member visits a dentist every six months for examinations and professional cleanings, it is important to maintain oral health between those visits.

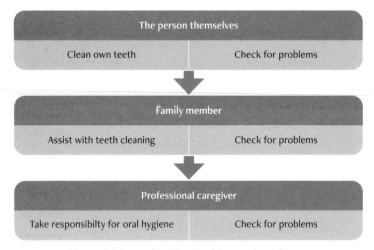

Figure 9.2 Procedure for checking teeth and gums and informally assessing oral health

The person themselves remains able to take care of their own teeth cleaning and knows when there may be problems. If they have tooth, gum or jaw pain or observe bleeding or swelling, they should notify a family member or make an appointment to see their dentist.

The family member assisting with teeth cleaning should encourage the person to clean their teeth and care for their mouth at least twice a day. Enable the individual to do as much for themselves as possible. Ensure that you also check for any early signs of tooth decay, damage to teeth or gum disease. If you feel there may be a problem, encourage the person to make an appointment with their dentist.

The professional caregiver taking responsibility for oral hygiene must carry out oral care at least twice daily and after the person has taken any medicine:

- Ensure that the person is in a comfortable position.

- Ensure that you can access their teeth and gums.

- Ensure that you wear surgical gloves.

- Communicate with the person at all times.

- Explain what you are doing and why.

- Clean the person's teeth in the way you have been trained (seek advice from the dentist or dental hygienist if you are unsure or if things have changed since you were trained).

- If the person wears dentures, clean them twice daily and ensure that the gums are clean too (at the beginning of this book we identified that one in ten older adults die from aspiration pneumonia, thus keeping the mouth clean of debris is massively important to oral hygiene).

- Check for any signs of pain and discomfort of the teeth and gums.

- Look for swollen gums or bleeding.

- Inform a dental health professional if you observe, or suspect, oral disease of any kind.

Remember that the sooner the intervention, the better the outcome.

Question 4

If I am to brush the teeth of a family member living with dementia, do I need to learn a special technique?

Seek advice from your dental professional as each individual is different. Some people require more assistance than others and there may be a special technique required. Always follow the instructions of the dental professional.

Question 5

What non-pharmacological strategies can I use to help my family member relax before visiting a dentist or carrying out oral hygiene with them?

Self-relaxation techniques can help relax people naturally. Try using the following prior to a visit to the dentist:

Ask the person to sit down and get comfortable. Feet firmly on the ground. In a soft, calm voice say:

Close your eyes and take five deep breaths. Relax. Imagine being on a beach. Feel the soft, warm grains of sand between your toes as you walk across the beach. Feel the warm breeze as it gently flows over your body. Feel the warmth from the sun as it shines onto your arms, back and legs. Relax. Breathe out and relax. Continue to focus on your breathing and sit by the edge of the water. Enjoy hearing the sounds of the waves lapping in and out. Listen to the music you can hear in the background. Relax. Relax.

The music you can play in the background is called *Weightless* by Marconi Union. Neuroscientists in the UK have determined that listening to *Weightless* resulted in a 65 per cent reduction in overall anxiety.

This is something you can repeat as many times as you need. It can also be done in the dental office waiting room.

References

Abbayya, K. Puthanakar, N.Y., Naduwinmani, S. and Chidambar, Y.S. (2015) 'Association between periodontitis and Alzheimer's disease.' *North American Journal of Medical Sciences*, 7(6) 241–246.

Evans, S. (2018, 4 January) NHS dentistry described as an 'international disgrace' in Daily Telegraph. Dentistry.co.uk. Available at: www.dentistry.co.uk/2018/01/04/nhs-dentistry-described-international-disgrace-daily-telegraph.

Garrard, C. (reviewed by Alexa Meara, MD) (2016) 'Rheumatoid arthritis and gum disease: what you need to know.' *Everyday Health*. Available at: www.everydayhealth.com/rheumatoid-arthritis/living-with/the-link-between-gum-disease-and-rheumatoid-arthritis.

Gupta, S., Pk, P. and Gupta, R. (2016) 'Necessity of oral health intervention in schizophrenic patients – A review.' *Nepal Journal of Epidemiology*, 6(4) 605–612.

Ilievski, V., Zuchowska, P.K., Green, S.J., Toth, P.T. *et al.* (2018) 'Chronic oral application of a periodontal pathogen results in brain inflammation, neurodegeneration and amyloid beta production in wild type mice.' *PLoS ONE*, 13(10) e0204941. doi:10.1371/journal.pone.0204941.

Lee, Y.T., Lee, H.C., Hu, C.J., Huang, L.K. *et al.* (2017) 'Periodontitis as a modifiable risk factor for dementia: A nationwide population-based cohort study.' *The Journal of the American Geriatrics Society*, 65(2) 301–305.

Manabe, T., Teramoto, S., Tamiya, N., Okochi, J. and Hizawa, N. (2015) 'Risk factors for aspiration pneumonia in older adults.' *PLoS One*, 10(10). Available at: https://core.ac.uk/download/pdf/56661447.pdf.

Nightingale, D. (2019) *A Clinician's Guide to Non-Pharmacological Dementia Therapies*. London and Philadelphia, PA: Jessica Kingsley Publishers.

Sabbagh, M. and MacMillan, B. (2012) *The Alzheimer's Prevention Cookbook: Recipes to Boost Brain Health*. New York, NY: Ten Speed Press.

Snowdon, D. (2001) *Aging with Grace: What the Nun Study Teaches Us About Leading Longer, Healthier, and More Meaningful Lives.* New York, NY: Bantam Books.

Telgi, R.L., Yadav, V., Telgi, C.R. and Boppana, N. (2013) 'In vivo dental plaque pH after consumption of dairy products.' *General Dentistry*, 61(3) 56–59.

Index